THE STROKE DIET COOKBOOK

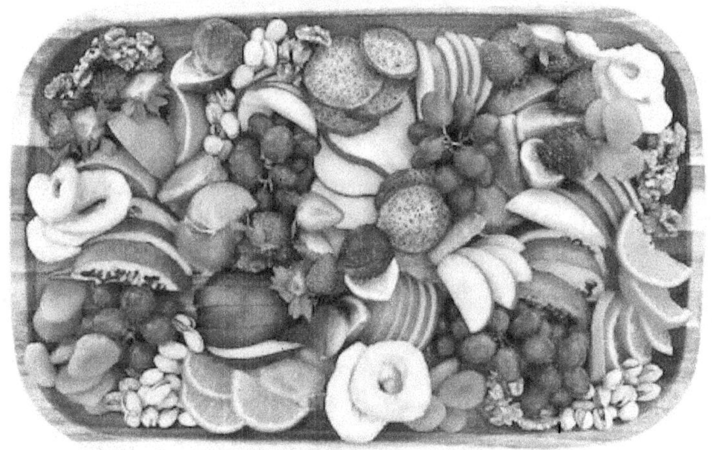

BY

DR. VICKIE STOCK

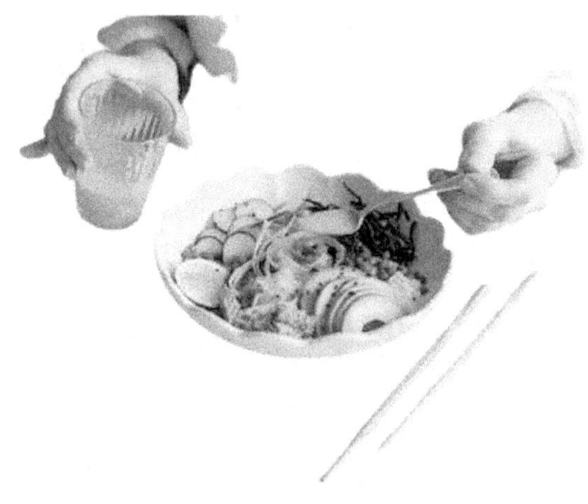

INTRODUCTION TO STROKE PREVENTION

Strokes stand as ominous threats that can alter lives in an instant. A stroke, often referred to as a "brain attack," occurs when blood flow to the brain is disrupted, leading to a cascade of debilitating consequences.

Recognizing the severity of strokes underscores the critical importance of preventive measures, a cornerstone in the realm of healthcare. Stroke prevention is not merely a response to a looming danger but a proactive commitment to preserving the delicate balance of well-being.

This journey begins with a deep understanding of the factors that contribute to stroke risk. Lifestyle choices, genetic predispositions, and underlying health conditions all play pivotal roles in shaping an individual's vulnerability to strokes.

The Introduction to Stroke Prevention seeks to unravel the intricate connections between these elements, fostering awareness that empowers individuals to take charge of their health destinies.

As we delve into the layers of stroke prevention, the central role of a healthy diet becomes evident. Nutrient-rich foods and mindful eating habits emerge as potent tools in fortifying the body against the onslaught of strokes.

The chapter explores the impact of essential elements like omega-3 fatty acids, antioxidants, and fiber on vascular health. It also sheds light on the significance of limiting sodium and unhealthy fats, steering readers towards choices that serve as shields against stroke risks.

Beyond dietary considerations, the introduction emphasizes the symbiotic relationship between diet and physical activity. Exercise emerges not just as a means of weight management but as a dynamic force that contributes significantly to overall cardiovascular health.

By understanding this connection, individuals can craft personalized strategies that seamlessly integrate physical activity into their daily routines, forging a holistic approach to stroke prevention.

CHAPTER ONE

The Importance of a Healthy Diet

In the symphony of well-being, the role of a healthy diet resonates as a powerful and harmonious melody, influencing every facet of our lives.

Beyond the conventional notions of weight management, a healthy diet stands as a cornerstone of preventive medicine, a shield against an array of maladies.

Nowhere is its significance more apparent than in the realm of stroke prevention, where dietary choices wield transformative powers, shaping the delicate balance between health and affliction.

A healthy diet is not merely a collection of nutritional components but a dynamic interplay of vitamins, minerals, antioxidants, and macronutrients that orchestrate the intricate dance of cellular functions.

At the forefront of the fight against strokes is the understanding that the food we consume is intricately linked to the health of our cardiovascular system. As arteries weave through our bodies like rivers, delivering life-sustaining oxygen and nutrients to the brain, the impact of diet on these vital conduits becomes undeniable.

High blood pressure, elevated cholesterol levels, and inflammation—precursors to strokes—are often direct consequences of dietary choices. The importance of a healthy diet in stroke prevention lies in its ability to modulate these risk factors.

Foods rich in omega-3 fatty acids, found in fatty fish like salmon and flaxseeds, emerge as defenders of cardiovascular health, reducing the risk of blood clots and promoting optimal blood flow to the brain.

Antioxidant-rich fruits and vegetables, vibrant in color and life, combat inflammation, mitigating the stress on blood vessels and fortifying the body's defense mechanisms.

Moreover, a healthy diet is a guardian of metabolic equilibrium, a regulator of weight and hormonal balance. Excess body weight, often a result of poor dietary choices, is a known contributor to diabetes—a condition that, in turn, elevates the risk of strokes. Through the prism of a healthy diet, individuals can recalibrate their relationship with food, forging a sustainable alliance that transcends the transient allure of fad diets and embraces a nourishing, long-term commitment to health.

Beyond the physical, the importance of a healthy diet extends to the realm of mental well-being. Nutrient-rich foods are not only fuel for the body but also sustenance for the brain.

The intricate network of neurons, the brain's messengers, relies on a diverse array of nutrients to function optimally. Studies suggest that diets high in antioxidants and omega-3 fatty acids may have cognitive benefits, further underscoring the holistic impact of a nutritious diet.

The importance of a healthy diet is a narrative of empowerment—a story where individuals wield the pen to script their own tales of well-being. It is an acknowledgment that the food on our plates is not merely a means of satiating hunger but a profound determinant of the quality and longevity of our lives.

As we navigate the complexities of dietary choices, let us embrace the significance of a healthy diet not as a prescription for deprivation but as a celebration of vitality—a key to unlocking the doors to a future where strokes are not just preventable but where health thrives as a vibrant and enduring legacy.

How Diet Affects Stroke Risk

Diet emerges as a linchpin, intricately woven into the fabric of our well-being. Nowhere is its impact more profound than in the realm of stroke risk.

The connection between what we eat and the likelihood of experiencing a stroke is a dynamic interplay of nutrients, lifestyle choices, and their intricate dance with our cardiovascular system.

Diet, in its essence, is a silent architect of our internal landscape. Its influence on stroke risk begins with its role in modulating key cardiovascular risk factors. High blood pressure, often regarded as the "silent killer," is a primary contributor to strokes.

Sodium-laden diets, prevalent in processed foods and excessive salt consumption, can elevate blood pressure, creating a turbulent environment within our arteries. The journey to understand how diet affects stroke risk is, therefore, a quest to decipher the intricate code of nutrients that can either soothe or disrupt this delicate equilibrium.

The detrimental impact of high cholesterol on our vascular health is another chapter in the narrative of diet and stroke risk. Diets rich in saturated and trans fats contribute to elevated levels of LDL cholesterol, commonly known as the "bad" cholesterol.

These cholesterol particles can accumulate in the arteries, forming plaques that may rupture and trigger a stroke. Conversely, diets emphasizing the consumption of heart-healthy fats, such as those found in avocados and olive oil, act as guardians, promoting optimal cholesterol levels and reducing the risk of atherosclerosis.

The sugar-laden landscape of modern diets also features prominently in the tale of stroke risk. Beyond its association with obesity and diabetes, excessive sugar intake may contribute to inflammation and oxidative stress—factors that fuel the development of arterial plaques.

Understanding how diet affects stroke risk involves peeling back the layers of hidden sugars and refined carbohydrates, revealing the potential harm lurking behind seemingly innocuous choices.

Yet, the narrative is not solely about avoidance; it's also about embracing the life-affirming properties of certain foods. Omega-3 fatty acids, abundant in fatty fish like salmon and walnuts, exhibit anti-inflammatory and anti-clotting effects, contributing to a vascular environment less prone to strokes.

Antioxidant-rich fruits and vegetables, with their vibrant hues, offer a protective shield against oxidative stress, promoting resilience in the face of potential stroke triggers.

In the grand tapestry of diet and stroke risk, the story extends beyond individual nutrients to encompass the broader spectrum of lifestyle choices. Physical inactivity, excess alcohol consumption, and smoking—all elements influenced by lifestyle and dietary habits—contribute significantly to stroke risk.

Understanding how diet affects stroke risk necessitates a holistic perspective, recognizing the interconnectedness of our choices and their profound impact on the health of our arteries and, consequently, our neurological well-being. As we unravel the intricate threads of this narrative, the overarching theme is one of empowerment.

It's a call to action, an invitation to wield the fork as a tool for health rather than a mere utensil for sustenance. The journey to mitigate stroke risk through dietary choices is a voyage into the heart of self-care, where mindful decisions ripple through the vascular system, shaping a future where strokes are not predetermined destinies but preventable outcomes of informed, nourishing choices.

Key Nutrients for Stroke Prevention

In the canvas of preventive healthcare, the spotlight on stroke prevention unveils a palette rich in essential nutrients that intricately shape the landscape of vascular well-being.

These key nutrients, with their unique abilities and synergies, become the architects of resilience against the looming threat of strokes. As we delve into the intricate tapestry of nutrition, a vivid portrait emerges—a story of empowerment through nourishment.

Omega-3 fatty acids, hailed as unsung heroes in the realm of cardiovascular health, take center stage in the saga of stroke prevention. Abundant in fatty fish like salmon, mackerel, and trout, as well as in flaxseeds and walnuts, these fatty acids offer a multifaceted defense.

Their anti-inflammatory properties soothe the intricate network of blood vessels, reducing the risk of plaque formation and blood clotting—two precursors to strokes.

Understanding the role of omega-3 fatty acids in stroke prevention invites individuals to embrace the richness of these foods, turning the dining table into a canvas for vascular well-being.

Antioxidants, like vigilant sentinels stationed within vibrant fruits and vegetables, add a burst of color to the narrative of stroke prevention. Vitamins C and E, along with a spectrum of phytochemicals, work in harmony to neutralize oxidative stress—the rust that threatens the integrity of our arterial walls.

Berries, citrus fruits, leafy greens, and nuts become not just culinary delights but essential tools in fortifying the body's defense against the oxidative triggers that may lead to strokes.

The story unfolds in every bite, where the vibrant hues signify not just flavor but a commitment to vascular health. Fiber, an unsung champion in the dietary arena, weaves its own narrative of stroke prevention.

Abundant in whole grains, legumes, fruits, and vegetables, fiber contributes to the maintenance of healthy blood pressure and cholesterol levels. Its soluble form acts like a sponge, absorbing cholesterol and ushering it out of the body, while its insoluble counterpart promotes digestive health.

In this tale of dietary choices, fiber becomes the silent guardian, fostering an environment within the body that resists the factors that may precipitate strokes.

Potassium, a mineral found in bananas, sweet potatoes, and leafy greens, steps onto the stage as a regulator of blood pressure—a key player in the stroke prevention saga.

Its ability to counterbalance the sodium in our diets contributes to the delicate dance of electrolytes, maintaining a harmonious fluid balance that eases the strain on our arteries.

Recognizing the importance of potassium in stroke prevention is an invitation to savor the natural richness of foods that hold this mineral, fostering a diet that nurtures not just taste buds but the intricate physiology of cardiovascular resilience.

Calcium and magnesium, often associated with bone health, also play pivotal roles in the orchestration of stroke prevention. Found in dairy products, nuts, and leafy greens, these minerals contribute to the stability of blood vessel walls and the regulation of blood pressure.

Their partnership with other key nutrients forms a holistic approach to vascular health, underscoring the interconnectedness of dietary choices in safeguarding against strokes.

As we immerse ourselves in the narrative of key nutrients for stroke prevention, the culinary realm transforms into a sanctuary of well-being. Each meal becomes an opportunity to fortify the body, a conscious act of nourishment that transcends the immediate gratification of taste to become a legacy of lasting health.

In the synergy of omega-3 fatty acids, antioxidants, fiber, potassium, calcium, and magnesium, we find not just nutrients but the protagonists in a tale of empowerment—a story where dietary choices become the compass guiding us toward a future where strokes are not merely feared but prevented through the mindful artistry of nutrition.

Foods to Include and Avoid in a Stroke Diet

The narrative of a stroke diet unfolds as a compelling story, where the protagonist—the careful selection of foods—becomes the guiding force in the quest for vascular resilience.

This culinary journey is not just about satisfying hunger; it is a strategic maneuver, a conscious choice that can tip the scales between health and the precipice of stroke risk. Let's explore the chapters of foods to include and avoid, each page turning towards a future where wellness is not just a goal but a lived reality.

➤ **Foods to Include:**

1. Colorful Fruits and Vegetables:

In the vibrant palette of nature lies an array of fruits and vegetables, each hue signaling a wealth of essential nutrients.

These colorful wonders are rich in antioxidants, vitamins, and minerals that fortify the body against inflammation and oxidative stress—the subtle adversaries that may lead to strokes.

Berries, citrus fruits, leafy greens, and cruciferous vegetables become not only culinary delights but also potent tools in the arsenal of stroke prevention.

2. Fatty Fish and Omega-3 Rich Foods:

The omega-3 fatty acids found in fatty fish like salmon, mackerel, and trout, as well as in flaxseeds and walnuts, take center stage in the narrative of vascular well-being.

These essential fats offer anti-inflammatory and anti-clotting benefits, creating a protective shield against the factors that may contribute to strokes. Including these foods in the diet is a flavorful commitment to cardiovascular health.

3. Whole Grains:

The unrefined goodness of whole grains, such as brown rice, quinoa, and oats, becomes the sturdy foundation of a stroke-preventive diet. Rich in fiber, vitamins, and minerals, whole grains contribute to stable blood pressure and cholesterol levels.

They offer sustained energy and satiety, turning meals into nourishing experiences that resonate beyond immediate gratification.

4. Healthy Fats:

Embracing sources of healthy fats, such as avocados, olive oil, and nuts, adds a layer of protection to the cardiovascular system.

These fats, in contrast to their saturated counterparts, contribute to optimal cholesterol levels and overall heart health. Drizzling olive oil over salads or enjoying a handful of nuts becomes a flavorful expression of dietary wisdom.

5. Lean Proteins:

Lean proteins, sourced from poultry, fish, legumes, and tofu, form the building blocks of a stroke-conscious diet. These proteins contribute to muscle health, metabolic balance, and overall satiety, creating a balanced and satisfying culinary landscape.

> ➤ **Foods to Avoid:**

1. Excessive Sodium:

The villain in the stroke prevention story often wears the cloak of excessive sodium. Processed foods, canned goods, and restaurant fare high in sodium can elevate blood pressure, increasing the risk of strokes.

Choosing fresh, whole foods and being mindful of sodium intake becomes a pivotal plot point in this dietary tale.

2. Saturated and Trans Fats:

The antagonists known as saturated and trans fats, lurking in fried foods, pastries, and processed snacks, threaten the cardiovascular harmony. Steering clear of these unhealthy fats is an essential chapter in the narrative of stroke prevention, making way for heart-healthy alternatives.

3. Excessive Sugar and Refined Carbohydrates:

The sweet seduction of excessive sugar and refined carbohydrates contributes to inflammation and metabolic imbalance. Limiting the intake of sugary beverages, candies, and white flour products becomes a conscious step towards maintaining vascular health.

4. Processed and Red Meats:

The protagonists in this dietary saga are lean proteins, not their processed or red counterparts. High intake of processed and red meats may contribute to unhealthy cholesterol levels and increase the risk of strokes.

Opting for lean protein sources, such as poultry and fish, reshapes the narrative towards a heart-friendly plot.

5. Alcohol and Caffeine in Moderation:

The subplot of alcohol and caffeine introduces moderation as the guiding principle. Excessive consumption may disrupt blood pressure and contribute to dehydration. Understanding the balance between enjoyment and limitation becomes an integral theme in crafting a stroke-conscious diet.

In stroke diet, each meal becomes a brushstroke on the canvas of health—a conscious creation that echoes through the corridors of vascular resilience.

The foods we choose to include and avoid are not just ingredients but narrative elements, shaping a story where strokes are not feared but prevented through the artistry of mindful, nourishing choices.

Dietary Considerations for Different Ages

In the symphony of life, our nutritional needs ebb and flow like the changing tides. From the tender beginnings of infancy to the seasoned wisdom of later years, each stage of life demands a unique dietary composition to support growth, vitality, and overall well-being. Understanding and embracing these dietary considerations for different ages is a key element in the pursuit of lifelong health and resilience.

Infancy and Early Childhood:

The opening chapter in the book of life, infancy, lays the foundation for future health. Breast milk or formula becomes the primary sustenance, providing the essential nutrients crucial for growth and development.

As children transition to solid foods, an exploration of nutrient-rich, age-appropriate options is pivotal. Iron-rich foods support cognitive development, while a variety of fruits and vegetables introduce a spectrum of vitamins and minerals. The emphasis on establishing healthy eating habits at this stage sets the tone for a lifetime of nutritional awareness.

Childhood and Adolescence:

As the curtain rises on childhood and adolescence, energy needs surge with the pace of growth spurts and increased physical activity. Whole grains, lean proteins, and a colorful array of fruits and vegetables take center stage.

Calcium and vitamin D play starring roles in bone health during these formative years. Encouraging a diverse and balanced diet becomes paramount, fostering a positive relationship with food that transcends the tumultuous adolescent years.

Young Adulthood:

The chapter of young adulthood unfolds with the pursuit of independence, and dietary choices play a pivotal role in maintaining vitality and preventing chronic diseases.

Nutrient-dense foods, including lean proteins, complex carbohydrates, and heart-healthy fats, form the cornerstone of a diet that supports a busy, active lifestyle. Building habits such as mindful eating and staying hydrated become integral components in this stage of life.

Middle Age:

Midlife marks a chapter where dietary considerations shift towards sustaining health and preventing age-related conditions. Nutrient needs remain high, but the focus expands to include heart health, bone density, and metabolic balance. Incorporating omega-3 fatty acids, fiber, and antioxidant-rich foods becomes crucial.

Mindful portion control and regular physical activity take precedence in navigating the challenges of metabolism and hormonal changes.

Later Years:

In the denouement of life's journey, dietary considerations evolve to address the changing needs of aging bodies. Adequate protein intake becomes imperative for muscle maintenance, while calcium and vitamin D continue to support bone health.

Emphasizing nutrient-dense foods becomes paramount, as caloric needs may decrease while the necessity for essential nutrients remains steadfast. Hydration and maintaining social connections through shared meals contribute to holistic well-being in the golden years.

Lifelong Principles:

Throughout this literary journey of dietary considerations, certain principles weave through every chapter. Moderation, balance, and variety emerge as timeless themes, transcending age. Mindful eating, staying hydrated, and adapting to individual needs underscore the importance of a flexible approach to nutrition that aligns with the unique requirements of each life stage.

The narrative of dietary considerations for different ages is a dynamic tale of adaptation and evolution. Just as characters evolve in a story, our nutritional needs metamorphose across the chapters of life.

Embracing these considerations is not a rigid script but a fluid dialogue with the body—a continuous dance that honors the ebb and flow of life's nutritional symphony.

Through this understanding, individuals can craft a dietary narrative that resonates with vitality, resilience, and the timeless pursuit of holistic well-being across the diverse landscapes of life.

Incorporating Physical Activity

The rhythmic dance between the human body and physical activity is a timeless narrative of health, vitality, and holistic well-being. From the tender steps of childhood play to the seasoned strides of later years, the importance of incorporating physical activity transcends age, weaving a narrative that resonates with the essence of a life well-lived.

Childhood and Adolescence: The Playful Prelude

In the opening chapters of life, physical activity takes the form of play—a spontaneous, joyful exploration that lays the groundwork for a lifetime of movement.

The playground becomes a canvas where coordination, balance, and social skills are painted into the developing tapestry of a child's well-being.

From organized sports to unstructured play, this stage sets the tone for a positive relationship with physical activity, fostering habits that extend far beyond the schoolyard.

Young Adulthood: The Energetic Flourish

As the curtain rises on young adulthood, physical activity evolves into a dynamic force that not only supports health but becomes an integral part of lifestyle.

The gym, sports, and outdoor adventures become outlets for the boundless energy characteristic of this stage. Beyond the pursuit of fitness, physical activity becomes a conduit for stress relief, a means of fostering mental well-being, and a social catalyst that strengthens connections.

Midlife: Navigating the Tempo

The middle chapters of life often bring a shifting tempo in the dance with physical activity. Career demands, family responsibilities, and time constraints can influence the rhythm.

Yet, this is a pivotal juncture where maintaining regular physical activity becomes not just a choice but a necessity. Activities that blend into daily routines, such as brisk walks, cycling, or yoga, take center stage.

The focus shifts towards sustainable practices that contribute to cardiovascular health, weight management, and overall resilience.

Later Years: The Graceful Waltz

In the later chapters, physical activity adopts the grace of a waltz—a gentle yet powerful expression of movement. Adaptability and inclusivity become the key themes.

Activities like swimming, tai chi, or low-impact exercises preserve joint health while enhancing balance and flexibility. The narrative of physical activity in the later years is a testament to the enduring benefits—maintaining independence, preventing chronic conditions, and fostering a sense of purpose and fulfillment.

Lifelong Principles: The Eternal Dance

Throughout the unfolding narrative of physical activity, certain principles remain timeless. Consistency emerges as a steadfast companion, transcending age and circumstance.

The significance of variety, whether in the form of different activities or adapting to changing abilities, underlines the versatility of the dance.

The synergy between physical activity and mental well-being becomes a harmonious duet, with each movement contributing to a symphony of holistic health.

CHAPTER TWO

Exercise and Its Impact on Stroke Prevention

Exercise emerges as a commanding maestro, directing a dynamic symphony of well-being. Its impact on stroke prevention transcends the boundaries of mere physical activity, weaving a narrative of resilience, vascular fortitude, and a symphony of physiological harmony.

Cardiovascular Resilience:

At the heart of exercise's role in stroke prevention lies its profound impact on cardiovascular health. Regular physical activity is akin to a rhythmic pulse, infusing vitality into the intricate network of blood vessels.

Aerobic exercises, such as brisk walking, running, cycling, and swimming, elevate the heart rate, promoting efficient blood flow and reducing the risk of hypertension—a major contributor to strokes.

This cardiovascular resilience becomes a shield, fortifying the arteries against the turbulence that may lead to stroke-related complications.

Blood Pressure Regulation:

Hypertension, often referred to as the "silent killer," is a potent precursor to strokes. Exercise, as a therapeutic intervention, becomes a stabilizing force in blood pressure regulation.

Engaging in moderate-intensity activities on a regular basis helps maintain healthy blood pressure levels. This harmonious balance is not just a momentary benefit; it resonates as a long-term investment in vascular well-being, mitigating one of the primary risk factors associated with strokes.

Weight Management and Metabolic Harmony:

Exercise unfurls its impact on stroke prevention through the lens of weight management and metabolic equilibrium. Physical activity contributes to calorie expenditure, helping individuals achieve and maintain a healthy weight.

Excess body weight is not just a cosmetic concern; it is a tangible risk factor for conditions such as diabetes and cardiovascular diseases, which amplify the likelihood of strokes.

The metabolic dance facilitated by exercise becomes a melody of prevention—a tune that promotes insulin sensitivity, lipid profile balance, and overall metabolic harmony.

Enhanced Blood Flow and Oxygenation:

The rhythm of exercise orchestrates enhanced blood flow and oxygenation to vital organs, including the brain. This increased circulation promotes the delivery of oxygen and nutrients to brain cells, fostering an environment of neurovascular resilience.

As the body engages in regular physical activity, the intricate network of blood vessels adapts, becoming more efficient and responsive—an evolutionary crescendo that echoes in reduced stroke risk.

Stress Reduction and Mental Well-being:

Beyond the physiological dimensions, exercise contributes to stroke prevention by addressing the intricate interplay between mental well-being and vascular health. Chronic stress, a silent contributor to strokes, finds a counterbalance in the stress-reducing effects of exercise.

The release of endorphins, often referred to as the "feel-good" hormones, creates a harmonious melody that not only uplifts mood but also contributes to a physiological environment less prone to the inflammation and tension that may lead to strokes.

Lifelong Impact:

The impact of exercise on stroke prevention is not a fleeting overture but a lifelong symphony. Its effects extend across the chapters of life, adapting to the evolving needs of individuals.

From the exuberant play of childhood to the measured steps of later years, exercise remains a steadfast companion—a narrative of vitality, resilience, and enduring well-being.

Exercise and its impact on stroke prevention is a profound composition, where each movement contributes to a harmonious melody of health.

Engaging in regular physical activity is not just a prescription; it is an ode to the resilient potential of the human body. As individuals participate in this dynamic symphony, they become not just spectators but active participants in the prevention of strokes—a collaborative effort where the maestro of exercise conducts a timeless performance of well-being.

Meal Planning Strategies: Crafting a Culinary Symphony for Health

Meal planning emerges as a beacon of order and health. It is not merely a pragmatic approach to nourishment but a culinary symphony—a thoughtful composition that orchestrates flavors, nutrition, and convenience into a harmonious tapestry of well-being.

1. Balancing Macronutrients:

At the heart of meal planning strategies is the artful balance of macronutrients—proteins, carbohydrates, and fats. Each meal becomes a canvas where these nutritional elements are thoughtfully distributed to provide sustained energy, satiety, and a comprehensive spectrum of essential nutrients.

Protein sources, such as lean meats, legumes, and tofu, form the cornerstone of a well-balanced plate, complemented by whole grains and an array of colorful vegetables.

2. Portion Control:

In the culinary symphony of health, portion control is a virtuoso performance. It involves understanding not just the nutritional composition of foods but also the appropriate serving sizes.

Meal planning strategies incorporate mindful portioning to avoid overconsumption, promoting a sense of satiety without unnecessary caloric excess.

This consideration extends beyond weight management; it fosters a mindful relationship with food, allowing individuals to savor each bite and listen to their body's hunger and fullness cues.

3. Creating Flavorful and Nutrient-Rich Meals:

The melody of meal planning resounds in the flavors and nutrient density of each dish. Embracing a variety of herbs and spices becomes a culinary crescendo, enhancing taste without relying on excessive salt or unhealthy fats.

The inclusion of nutrient-rich ingredients, such as leafy greens, colorful vegetables, and whole grains, adds depth to the composition, ensuring that each meal is not just a source of sustenance but a celebration of vibrant, wholesome flavors.

4. Healthy Cooking Techniques:

The culinary repertoire of meal planning extends to the techniques employed in the kitchen. Baking, grilling, steaming, and sautéing become the instruments through which flavors are coaxed and textures are perfected.

These methods preserve the nutritional integrity of ingredients, avoiding the pitfalls of excessive oil or calorie-dense cooking practices. The result is a symphony of meals that are both health-conscious and culinary delights.

5. Building a Stroke-Friendly Pantry:

Meal planning strategies also extend to the meticulous curation of a stroke-friendly pantry. This involves stocking up on whole grains, legumes, lean proteins, and heart-healthy oils.

Canned and frozen options, carefully selected for their nutritional value and low sodium content, become the supporting cast.

By cultivating a pantry that aligns with stroke prevention principles, meal planning becomes a seamless and health-conscious endeavor.

6. Adapting for Individual Needs:

The beauty of meal planning lies in its adaptability to individual preferences, dietary restrictions, and health considerations.

Whether tailoring meals for specific medical conditions, accommodating different ages, or catering to personal taste preferences, effective meal planning strategies are versatile. They allow individuals to navigate the vast culinary landscape while adhering to the principles of nutrition and health.

7. Considering Social and Cultural Influences:

In the grand composition of meal planning, social and cultural influences provide the rich undertones that make each meal unique.

Strategies take into account the diverse traditions, culinary heritage, and communal aspects of dining. This ensures that meal planning is not a rigid directive but a flexible and inclusive practice that resonates with the diverse tastes and preferences of individuals and communities.

Causes Of Stroke, Types of Stroke, Signs and Symptoms Of Stroke

Causes of Stroke:

A stroke, often referred to as a "brain attack," occurs when there is a disruption in blood flow to the brain, leading to damage or death of brain cells. The causes of stroke can be categorized into two main types: ischemic and hemorrhagic.

Ischemic Stroke:

> **Thrombotic Stroke:** Caused by a blood clot (thrombus) that forms in one of the arteries supplying blood to the brain.

> **Embolic Stroke:** Arises when a blood clot or other debris forms elsewhere in the body and travels to the brain, blocking a blood vessel.

Hemorrhagic Stroke:

> **Intracerebral Hemorrhage:** Occurs when a blood vessel within the brain ruptures, leading to bleeding and damage to surrounding brain tissue.

➢ **Subarachnoid Hemorrhage:** Involves bleeding into the space surrounding the brain, usually caused by the rupture of an aneurysm.

Contributing Factors to Stroke Risk:

Hypertension (High Blood Pressure): The leading cause of strokes.

Atherosclerosis: Build-up of plaque in arteries, narrowing or blocking blood flow.

Heart Conditions: Atrial fibrillation, heart valve disorders, and other cardiac issues can increase stroke risk.

Diabetes: Uncontrolled diabetes can damage blood vessels, contributing to stroke risk.

Smoking: Increases the likelihood of blood clot formation and atherosclerosis.

Obesity and Sedentary Lifestyle: Lack of physical activity and excess weight are risk factors.

Age and Gender: Stroke risk increases with age, and men are generally at higher risk than women.

Types of Stroke:

Ischemic Stroke:

- ➤ **Thrombotic Stroke**: Caused by a clot forming in a blood vessel supplying the brain.
- ➤ **Embolic Stroke:** Results from an embolus (a traveling clot) blocking a blood vessel in the brain.

Hemorrhagic Stroke:

- ➤ **Intracerebral Hemorrhage:** Occurs when a blood vessel within the brain ruptures.
- ➤ **Subarachnoid Hemorrhage:** Involves bleeding into the space surrounding the brain.

Signs and Symptoms of Stroke:

Recognizing the signs and symptoms of a stroke is crucial for seeking immediate medical attention, as prompt intervention can minimize damage. The common acronym FAST helps identify warning signs:

➢ **Face Drooping:**

Sudden numbness or weakness, especially on one side of the face. The person may struggle to smile, and their mouth or eye may droop.

➢ **Arm Weakness:**

Sudden numbness or weakness in one arm. If the person tries to raise both arms, one arm may drift downward.

➢ **Speech Difficulty:**

Slurred speech or difficulty speaking. The person may be unable to articulate words or phrases coherently.

➢ **Time to Call Emergency Services:**

If any of the above signs are observed, it's crucial to call emergency services immediately. Time is of the essence in stroke treatment.

Additional symptoms may include sudden severe headache, trouble walking, dizziness, and loss of coordination.

Strokes are complex events with varied causes, types, and manifestations. Recognizing the risk factors, understanding the types of strokes, and being aware of the signs and symptoms empower individuals to take prompt action and seek medical help, potentially preventing or minimizing the impact of a stroke on their health.

The Benefits of a Stroke Diet

A stroke diet is more than a prescription for preventing strokes; it is a culinary roadmap that navigates towards a future of robust health and vitality. Crafted with precision, this diet offers a plethora of benefits that extend beyond mere stroke prevention, influencing the entire spectrum of well-being.

1. Cardiovascular Health:

A stroke diet places a spotlight on cardiovascular health, acting as a guardian for the intricate network of blood vessels that nourish the body.

By emphasizing foods rich in omega-3 fatty acids, antioxidants, and fiber, the diet contributes to optimal blood flow, reduces inflammation, and addresses risk factors such as high blood pressure and cholesterol levels.

These benefits create a resilient cardiovascular system, lowering the likelihood of strokes while promoting heart health.

2. Blood Pressure Regulation:

Hypertension, a silent contributor to strokes, often finds its roots in dietary choices. A stroke diet strategically incorporates nutrients known to regulate blood pressure.

Reduced sodium intake, coupled with an abundance of potassium from fruits, vegetables, and whole grains, creates an optimal balance that supports healthy blood pressure levels. This regulatory effect not only aids in stroke prevention but fosters overall cardiovascular well-being.

3. Weight Management:

Excess body weight is a significant risk factor for strokes. A stroke diet embraces the principles of weight management through the promotion of nutrient-dense, low-calorie foods.

By prioritizing whole grains, lean proteins, and a colorful array of fruits and vegetables, the diet becomes a tool for maintaining a healthy weight.

This, in turn, mitigates the risk of conditions such as diabetes and obesity, further reducing the likelihood of strokes.

4. Antioxidant Defense Against Inflammation:

Antioxidants, found abundantly in fruits and vegetables, play a pivotal role in the stroke diet's arsenal against inflammation—the subtle precursor to strokes. These powerful compounds neutralize free radicals, reducing oxidative stress on blood vessels.

By infusing the body with antioxidants, the diet becomes a shield that fortifies against the inflammatory cascade, fostering an environment of resilience within the vascular system.

5. Improved Cognitive Function:

Beyond the physical, a stroke diet exhibits benefits for cognitive function. Omega-3 fatty acids, prevalent in fatty fish like salmon, are associated with cognitive health. T

he inclusion of these fats, along with other brain-boosting nutrients like vitamins and minerals, becomes a proactive measure in preserving cognitive function and reducing the risk of cognitive decline—a facet that aligns seamlessly with the overarching goal of well-being.

6. Adaptability Across Ages:

One of the remarkable aspects of a stroke diet is its adaptability across different ages. Whether catering to the developmental needs of children, supporting the energetic lifestyles of young adults, or addressing the specific considerations of older individuals, the diet's principles remain flexible. It transforms into a lifelong ally, adapting to the evolving nutritional requirements of individuals at various stages of life.

7. Holistic Nutritional Benefits:

At its essence, a stroke diet is not a restrictive set of guidelines; it is a celebration of vibrant, nourishing foods. Rich in vitamins, minerals, and a spectrum of nutrients, the diet becomes a symphony of flavors and textures that go beyond prevention.

It fosters a holistic approach to nutrition, encouraging individuals to savor the culinary delights that contribute to overall well-being.

CHAPTER THREE

Healthy Stroke Diet Recipes

Breakfast

1. Oatmeal with Berries and Almonds

Ingredients:

Rolled oats

Mixed berries (strawberries, blueberries, raspberries)

Almonds, chopped

Honey

Instructions:

Cook oats according to package instructions.

Top with mixed berries, chopped almonds, and a drizzle of honey.

Preparation Time: 10 minutes

2. Whole Wheat Toast with Avocado and Tomato

Ingredients:

Whole wheat bread

Avocado, mashed

Tomato slices

Salt and pepper

Instructions:

Toast the whole wheat bread.

Spread mashed avocado on the toast and top with tomato slices.

Season with salt and pepper.

Preparation Time: 5 minutes

3. Greek Yogurt Parfait

Ingredients:

Greek yogurt

Granola

Mixed fresh fruits (e.g., banana slices, berries)

Instructions:

Layer Greek yogurt with granola and mixed fruits.

Repeat layers.

Preparation Time: 7 minutes

4. Vegetable Omelette

Ingredients:

Eggs

Bell peppers, diced

Spinach

Tomatoes, chopped

Instructions:

Whisk eggs and pour into a heated non-stick pan.

Add diced bell peppers, spinach, and tomatoes.

Cook until eggs are set, then fold in half.

Preparation Time: 15 minutes

5. Smoothie Bowl

Ingredients:

Frozen mixed berries

Banana

Greek yogurt

Chia seeds

Instructions:

Blend berries, banana, and yogurt until smooth.

Pour into a bowl and top with chia seeds.

Preparation Time: 5 minutes

6. Quinoa Breakfast Bowl

Ingredients:

Cooked quinoa

Almond milk

Pecans

Dried apricots, chopped

Instructions:

Mix cooked quinoa with almond milk.

Top with pecans and dried apricots.

Preparation Time: 10 minutes

7. Whole Grain Pancakes

Ingredients:

Whole grain pancake mix

Fresh fruit (e.g., berries, sliced banana)

Maple syrup (optional)

Instructions:

Prepare pancakes according to the mix instructions.

Top with fresh fruit and a drizzle of maple syrup.

Preparation Time: 15 minutes

8. Chia Seed Pudding

Ingredients:

Chia seeds

Almond milk

Vanilla extract

Sliced almonds

Instructions:

Mix chia seeds, almond milk, and vanilla extract.

Refrigerate overnight, then top with sliced almonds.

Preparation Time: 5 minutes (plus overnight soaking)

9. Cottage Cheese with Pineapple

Ingredients:

Low-fat cottage cheese

Fresh pineapple chunks

Mint leaves for garnish

Instructions:

Combine cottage cheese and fresh pineapple chunks.

Garnish with mint leaves.

Preparation Time: 5 minutes

10. Smoked Salmon and Whole Grain Bagel

Ingredients:

Whole grain bagel

Smoked salmon

Cream cheese

Capers

Instructions:

Toast the whole grain bagel.

Spread cream cheese, top with smoked salmon, and sprinkle capers.

Preparation Time: 8 minutes

11. Fruit Salad with Mint

Ingredients:

Mixed fresh fruits (e.g., melon, grapes, kiwi)

Fresh mint leaves

Lime juice

Instructions:

Chop fruits and toss with fresh mint leaves.

Drizzle with lime juice.

Preparation Time: 10 minutes

12. Spinach and Feta Breakfast Wrap

Ingredients:

Whole grain wrap

Eggs, scrambled

Spinach

Feta cheese

Instructions:

Fill a whole grain wrap with scrambled eggs, spinach, and crumbled feta.

Roll and enjoy.

Preparation Time: 12 minutes

13. Peanut Butter Banana Toast

Ingredients:

Whole grain bread

Peanut butter

Banana slices

Instructions:

Toast whole grain bread.

Spread peanut butter and top with banana slices.

Preparation Time: 5 minutes

14. Mushroom and Spinach Frittata

Ingredients:

Eggs

Mushrooms, sliced

Spinach

Parmesan cheese

Instructions:

Whisk eggs and pour into a heated oven-safe pan.

Add sliced mushrooms and spinach, sprinkle with Parmesan.

Bake until eggs are set.

Preparation Time: 20 minutes

15. Brown Rice Porridge

Ingredients:

Cooked brown rice

Almond milk

Cinnamon

Sliced almonds

Instructions:

Mix cooked brown rice with almond milk and a dash of cinnamon.

Top with sliced almonds.

Preparation Time: 10 minutes

Lunch

1. Grilled Salmon Salad

Ingredients:

Salmon fillets

Mixed greens

Cherry tomatoes

Cucumber

Olive oil

Lemon juice

Salt and pepper

Instructions:

Season salmon with salt and pepper.

Grill salmon until cooked.

Toss mixed greens, cherry tomatoes, and cucumber.

Top salad with grilled salmon.

Drizzle with olive oil and lemon juice.

Preparation Time: 20 minutes

2. Quinoa and Vegetable Stir-Fry

Ingredients:

Quinoa

Broccoli

Bell peppers

Carrots

Snap peas

Soy sauce

Garlic

Sesame oil

Instructions:

Cook quinoa according to package instructions.

Stir-fry vegetables in sesame oil and garlic.

Add cooked quinoa and soy sauce.

Mix well until heated through.

Preparation Time: 25 minutes

3. Turkey and Avocado Wrap

Ingredients:

Whole-grain tortilla

Sliced turkey breast

Avocado

Lettuce

Tomato

Greek yogurt

Instructions:

Lay out tortilla and layer with turkey, avocado, lettuce, and tomato.

Spread Greek yogurt.

Roll up the wrap tightly.

Preparation Time: 15 minutes

4. Lentil and Vegetable Soup

Ingredients:

Lentils

Carrots

Celery

Onion

Garlic

Vegetable broth

Spinach

Instructions:

Sauté onion and garlic in a pot.

Add carrots, celery, lentils, and vegetable broth.

Simmer until lentils are tender.

Stir in spinach before serving.

Preparation Time: 30 minutes

5. Baked Chicken with Sweet Potato

Ingredients:

Chicken breast

Sweet potatoes

Olive oil

Rosemary

Garlic powder

Salt and pepper

Instructions:

Preheat oven to 400°F (200°C).

Rub chicken with olive oil, rosemary, garlic powder, salt, and pepper.

Place chicken and sliced sweet potatoes on a baking sheet.

Bake until chicken is cooked through and sweet potatoes are tender.

Preparation Time: 40 minutes

6. Shrimp and Vegetable Skewers

Ingredients:

Shrimp

Zucchini

Cherry tomatoes

Red onion

Olive oil

Lemon juice

Italian seasoning

Instructions:

Thread shrimp, zucchini, tomatoes, and onion onto skewers.

Mix olive oil, lemon juice, and Italian seasoning.

Brush skewers with the mixture.

Grill until shrimp is opaque.

Preparation Time: 25 minutes

7. Spinach and Feta Stuffed Chicken

Ingredients:

Chicken breast

Spinach

Feta cheese

Garlic

Olive oil

Salt and pepper

Instructions:

Preheat oven to 375°F (190°C).

Sauté spinach and garlic in olive oil until wilted.

Cut a pocket into each chicken breast.

Stuff with spinach and feta mixture.

Bake until chicken is cooked through.

Preparation Time: 35 minutes

8. Quinoa Salad with Chickpeas

Ingredients:

Quinoa

Chickpeas

Cucumber

Red bell pepper

Red onion

Feta cheese

Olive oil

Lemon juice

Instructions:

Cook quinoa according to package instructions.

Mix quinoa with chickpeas, cucumber, bell pepper, and red onion.

Crumble feta cheese on top.

Drizzle with olive oil and lemon juice.

Preparation Time: 30 minutes

9. Egg Salad Lettuce Wraps

Ingredients:

Hard-boiled eggs

Greek yogurt

Mustard

Celery

Lettuce leaves

Instructions:

Chop hard-boiled eggs and celery.

Mix with Greek yogurt and mustard.

Spoon onto lettuce leaves to make wraps.

Preparation Time: 15 minutes

10. Vegetable and Tofu Stir-Fry

Ingredients:

Tofu

Broccoli

Snow peas

Carrots

Bell peppers

Soy sauce

Ginger

Garlic

Instructions:

Press tofu to remove excess water and cut into cubes.

Stir-fry tofu and vegetables in soy sauce, ginger, and garlic.

Cook until vegetables are tender.

Preparation Time: 25 minutes

11. Mediterranean Quinoa Bowl

Ingredients:

Quinoa

Chickpeas

Cherry tomatoes

Cucumber

Kalamata olives

Feta cheese

Olive oil

Lemon juice

Instructions:

Cook quinoa according to package instructions.

Combine quinoa with chickpeas, tomatoes, cucumber, olives, and feta.

Drizzle with olive oil and lemon juice.

Preparation Time: 30 minutes

12. Baked Cod with Lemon and Herbs

Ingredients:

Cod fillets

Lemon

Fresh herbs (such as parsley or dill)

Olive oil

Garlic

Salt and pepper

Instructions:

Preheat oven to 400°F (200°C).

Place cod fillets in a baking dish.

Drizzle with olive oil, lemon juice, and sprinkle with herbs, garlic, salt, and pepper.

Bake until fish flakes easily.

Preparation Time: 25 minutes

13. Turkey and Vegetable Skillet

Ingredients:

Ground turkey

Bell peppers

Zucchini

Onion

Tomato sauce

Italian seasoning

Olive oil

Instructions:

Brown ground turkey in olive oil.

Add chopped vegetables and cook until tender.

Stir in tomato sauce and Italian seasoning.

Simmer until flavors meld.

Preparation Time: 30 minutes

14. Roasted Vegetable Wrap

Ingredients:

Assorted vegetables (e.g., bell peppers, zucchini, eggplant)

Whole-grain tortilla

Hummus

Spinach leaves

Instructions:

Toss vegetables in olive oil and roast until tender.

Spread hummus on a tortilla.

Add roasted vegetables and spinach.

Roll into a wrap.

Preparation Time: 35 minutes

15. Sweet Potato and Black Bean Bowl

Ingredients:

Sweet potatoes

Black beans

Corn

Avocado

Salsa

Cilantro

Lime

Instructions:

Roast sweet potatoes until tender.

Combine with black beans, corn, diced avocado, salsa, and cilantro.

Squeeze lime over the top.

Preparation Time: 40 minutes

Dinner

1. Grilled Salmon with Quinoa and Roasted Vegetables

Ingredients:

Salmon fillets

Quinoa

Assorted vegetables (e.g., bell peppers, zucchini, cherry tomatoes)

Olive oil

Lemon

Salt and pepper

Instructions:

Cook quinoa according to package instructions.

Marinate salmon with olive oil, lemon juice, salt, and pepper.

Grill salmon until cooked through.

Roast vegetables in the oven with olive oil, salt, and pepper.

Serve salmon over a bed of quinoa with roasted vegetables.

2. Chicken and Vegetable Stir-Fry

Ingredients:

Chicken breast, thinly sliced

Broccoli florets

Carrots, julienned

Bell peppers, sliced

Soy sauce

Ginger and garlic, minced

Brown rice

Instructions:

Stir-fry chicken until cooked through.

Add vegetables and stir-fry until crisp-tender.

Mix in soy sauce, ginger, and garlic.

Serve over brown rice.

3. Lentil and Vegetable Soup

Ingredients:

Green lentils

Carrots, diced

Celery, chopped

Onion, diced

Low-sodium vegetable broth

Spinach leaves

Garlic, minced

Instructions:

Saute onions and garlic until softened.

Add lentils, carrots, celery, and vegetable broth.

Simmer until lentils are tender.

Stir in spinach before serving.

4. Baked Cod with Sweet Potato Mash

Ingredients:

Cod fillets

Sweet potatoes, peeled and cubed

Greek yogurt

Dill, chopped

Olive oil

Lemon

Instructions:

Bake cod with olive oil and lemon until flaky.

Boil sweet potatoes until tender, then mash with Greek yogurt and dill.

Serve cod over sweet potato mash.

5. Quinoa Salad with Chickpeas and vegetables

Ingredients:

Quinoa

Chickpeas, drained and rinsed

Cherry tomatoes, halved

Cucumber, diced

Feta cheese

Olive oil and balsamic vinegar

Instructions:

Cook quinoa according to package instructions.

Mix quinoa with chickpeas, tomatoes, cucumber, and feta.

Drizzle with olive oil and balsamic vinegar.

6. Turkey and Vegetable Skewers

Ingredients:

Turkey breast, cut into chunks

Cherry tomatoes

Bell peppers, cut into squares

Olive oil

Italian seasoning

Garlic powder

Instructions:

Thread turkey, tomatoes, and peppers onto skewers.

Brush with olive oil and sprinkle with Italian seasoning and garlic powder.

Grill until turkey is cooked through.

7. Spinach and Mushroom Stuffed Chicken Breast

Ingredients:

Chicken breasts

Spinach

Mushrooms, chopped

Low-fat mozzarella cheese

Garlic powder

Olive oil

Instructions:

Saute mushrooms and spinach in olive oil until wilted.

Slice a pocket into chicken breasts and stuff with the spinach and mushroom mixture.

Bake until chicken is cooked, topping with mozzarella in the last few minutes.

8. Vegetable and Shrimp Stir-Fry with Brown Rice

Ingredients:

Shrimp, peeled and deveined

Broccoli florets

Snap peas

Carrots, sliced

Brown rice

Low-sodium soy sauce

Sesame oil

Instructions:

Cook shrimp in sesame oil until pink.

Add vegetables and stir-fry until tender.

Mix in soy sauce and serve over brown rice.

9. Quinoa and Black Bean Bowl

Ingredients:

Quinoa

Black beans, drained and rinsed

Avocado, sliced

Corn kernels

Lime juice

Cilantro, chopped

Instructions:

Cook quinoa according to package instructions.

Mix quinoa with black beans, avocado, and corn.

Squeeze lime juice over the bowl and garnish with cilantro.

10. Roasted Vegetable and Chicken Wrap

Ingredients:

Whole wheat wraps

Grilled chicken strips

Roasted vegetables (zucchini, bell peppers, onions)

Hummus

Spinach leaves

Instructions:

Lay out wraps and spread a layer of hummus.

Add chicken, roasted vegetables, and spinach.

Roll up and serve.

11. Sweet Potato and Black Bean Chili

Ingredients:

Sweet potatoes, diced

Black beans, drained and rinsed

Diced tomatoes

Chili powder

Cumin

Onion, diced

Instructions:

Saute onions until softened.

Add sweet potatoes, black beans, tomatoes, and spices.

Simmer until sweet potatoes are tender.

12. Lemon Herb Baked Tilapia with Quinoa

Ingredients:

Tilapia fillets

Lemon juice

Fresh herbs (such as thyme and parsley)

Quinoa

Olive oil

Instructions:

Preheat oven and bake tilapia with lemon juice and herbs.

Cook quinoa according to package instructions.

Serve tilapia over a bed of quinoa.

13. Turkey and Vegetable Skillet

Ingredients:

Ground turkey

Bell peppers, diced

Zucchini, sliced

Onion, chopped

Italian seasoning

Tomato sauce

Instructions:

Cook ground turkey in a skillet until browned.

Add vegetables and Italian seasoning, cook until tender.

Stir in tomato sauce and simmer.

14. Brown Rice and Vegetable Casserole

Ingredients:

Brown rice

Mixed vegetables (peas, carrots, corn)

Chicken broth

Parmesan cheese

Garlic powder

Onion, diced

Instructions:

Mix brown rice, vegetables, chicken broth, Parmesan, garlic powder, and diced onion in a casserole dish.

Bake until rice is cooked and vegetables are tender.

15. Mediterranean Chickpea Salad

Ingredients:

Chickpeas, drained and rinsed

Cherry tomatoes, halved

Cucumber, diced

Kalamata olives, sliced

Feta cheese

Olive oil and balsamic vinegar

Instructions:

Combine chickpeas, tomatoes, cucumber, olives, and feta in a bowl.

Drizzle with olive oil and balsamic vinegar, toss gently.

Snack

1. Greek Yogurt Parfait

Ingredients:

1 cup low-fat Greek yogurt

1/2 cup fresh berries

1 tablespoon honey

2 tablespoons chopped nuts (e.g., almonds or walnuts)

Instructions:

In a glass, layer Greek yogurt, fresh berries, and chopped nuts.

Drizzle honey on top.

Serve chilled.

Preparation Time: 5 minutes

2. Hummus with Veggie Sticks

Ingredients:

1/2 cup hummus

Carrot and cucumber sticks for dipping

Instructions:

Place hummus in a bowl.

Arrange veggie sticks for dipping.

Preparation Time: 5 minutes

3. Oatmeal Banana Cookies

Ingredients:

1 cup rolled oats

2 ripe bananas, mashed

1/4 cup chopped nuts

1 teaspoon vanilla extract

Instructions:

Preheat oven to 350°F (175°C).

Mix oats, mashed bananas, nuts, and vanilla.

Drop spoonfuls onto a baking sheet and bake for 12-15 minutes.

Preparation Time: 20 minutes (including baking time)

4. Avocado Toast

Ingredients:

1 slice whole-grain bread

1/2 ripe avocado

Pinch of salt and pepper

Optional: Cherry tomatoes for topping

Instructions:

Toast the bread slice.

Mash the avocado and spread it on the toast.

Sprinkle with salt and pepper, and top with cherry tomatoes if desired.

Preparation Time: 10 minutes

5. Cottage Cheese and Pineapple Bowl

Ingredients:

1/2 cup low-fat cottage cheese

1/2 cup fresh pineapple chunks

Instructions:

Mix cottage cheese and pineapple in a bowl.

Enjoy!

Preparation Time: 5 minutes

6. Smoothie Bowl

Ingredients:

1 cup frozen berries

1/2 banana

1/2 cup low-fat yogurt

1 tablespoon chia seeds

Instructions:

Blend berries, banana, and yogurt until smooth.

Pour into a bowl and sprinkle with chia seeds.

Preparation Time: 7 minutes

7. Rice Cake with Almond Butter

Ingredients:

1 rice cake

1 tablespoon almond butter

Instructions:

Spread almond butter on the rice cake.

Serve and enjoy.

Preparation Time: 3 minutes

8. Vegetable and Quinoa Salad

Ingredients:

1/2 cup cooked quinoa

Assorted chopped vegetables (bell peppers, cucumber, cherry tomatoes)

Olive oil and lemon dressing

Instructions:

Mix quinoa and vegetables.

Drizzle with olive oil and lemon dressing.

Preparation Time: 15 minutes

9. Apple Slices with Peanut Butter

Ingredients:

1 apple, sliced

2 tablespoons peanut butter

Instructions:

Spread peanut butter on apple slices.

Serve and enjoy.

Preparation Time: 5 minutes

10. Chia Seed Pudding

Ingredients:

2 tablespoons chia seeds

1/2 cup almond milk

1/2 teaspoon vanilla extract

Fresh berries for topping

Instructions:

Mix chia seeds, almond milk, and vanilla extract.

Refrigerate for a few hours or overnight.

Top with fresh berries before serving.

Preparation Time: 5 minutes (plus chilling time)

11. Turkey and Cheese Roll-ups

Ingredients:

Sliced turkey breast

Low-fat cheese slices

Whole grain tortilla

Instructions:

Place turkey and cheese on the tortilla.

Roll up and slice into bite-sized pieces.

Preparation Time: 8 minutes

12. Edamame Snack

Ingredients:

1 cup edamame (steamed)

Sea salt for sprinkling

Instructions:

Steam edamame according to package instructions.

Sprinkle with sea salt.

Preparation Time: 10 minutes

13. Whole Grain Crackers with Tuna Salad

Ingredients:

Whole grain crackers

Tuna salad (canned tuna, Greek yogurt, celery, and seasonings)

Instructions:

Top crackers with tuna salad.

Preparation Time: 10 minutes

14. Sliced Mango with Chili-Lime Seasoning

Ingredients:

1 ripe mango, sliced

Chili-lime seasoning

Instructions:

Sprinkle mango slices with chili-lime seasoning.

Preparation Time: 5 minutes

15. Cucumber and Cottage Cheese Bites

Ingredients:

Sliced cucumber rounds

Low-fat cottage cheese

Fresh dill for garnish

Instructions:

Top cucumber slices with cottage cheese.

Garnish with fresh dill. Preparation Time: 8 minutes

CONCLUSION

This stroke-friendly diet cookbook provides a diverse array of delicious and nutritious snack options tailored to support individuals on their journey to recovery and overall well-being.

Each recipe is thoughtfully crafted with a focus on incorporating wholesome ingredients, essential nutrients, and flavors that cater to both health and palate. Remember, the key to a successful stroke diet lies in balance, moderation, and individualized preferences.

Maintaining a healthy diet after a stroke is not only about nourishing the body but also about savoring the joy of eating. These recipes aim to make the dietary transition enjoyable, offering a variety of choices that can be easily integrated into daily life.

As always, it's crucial to consult with healthcare professionals or dietitians to ensure that the recipes align with specific dietary requirements and individual health conditions.

By embracing these stroke-friendly snacks, individuals can embark on a culinary journey that promotes healing, vitality, and the overall pursuit of a healthier lifestyle.

May this cookbook serve as a helpful guide, encouraging everyone to savor the goodness of wholesome ingredients and savor the taste of well-being. Here's to your health and the joy of nourishing both body and spirit through the power of mindful eating.